SQUAMOUS CELL CARCINOMA

A Comprehensive Strategy for the Management of Squamous Cell Carcinoma: A Lifestyle Guide to Dermatological Wellness

CHAD BRUNO

Table of Contents

Introductory...................................4

CHAPTER ONE 7

Causal Variables......................7

Symptoms and Indicators..........12

CHAPTER TWO 18

Diagnose and Classify...............18

Choices in Medical Care.............23

CHAPTER THREE 30

Prediction and Treatment 30

Safety and Security Measures 36

CHAPTER FOUR 44

Adjusting to a New Health Status
....44

Conclusion 51

THE END...................................54

Introductory

Squamous cell carcinoma (SCC) is a malignant neoplasm that begins in the flat, thin squamous cells that line the epidermis of the skin and the respiratory tract, as well as the oral cavity, pharynx, and cervix. Squamous cell carcinoma (SCC) is a kind of skin cancer that can develop on any part of the body.

• Malignant tumors emerge when this type of cancer develops as a result of the unchecked proliferation of squamous cells. The risk of developing SCC increases with cumulative sun exposure, and the condition is most commonly found on sun-exposed parts of the body, including the face, ears, neck, scalp, and backs of the hands. It's not limited to only the tongue and palate, either.

Early detection and treatment of squamous cell carcinoma greatly improves the chances of a successful recovery. Tumor removal surgery, radiation therapy, chemotherapy, and targeted therapy may all be alternatives. Patients with SCC would benefit greatly from early discovery and treatment, therefore it's crucial that they keep a close eye on their skin and visit a doctor if they notice any suspicious lesions or changes.

CHAPTER ONE
Causal Variables

Several variables may increase or decrease a person's vulnerability to developing squamous cell carcinoma (SCC). However, just because you have one or more of these risk factors doesn't mean you'll definitely have SCC. Squamous cell carcinoma risk factors often include:

1. Ultraviolet (UV) Exposure: Prolonged and recurrent exposure to UV radiation from the sun and tanning beds is a key risk factor for SCC. Spending a lot of time in the sun without proper protection puts you at a higher risk for skin cancer.

2. Fair Complexion: People with fair or pale complexion are at higher risk since they have less natural protection against UV rays.

3. Although SCC can develop at any age, it is more common in people over the age of 60.

4. A history of melanoma or another form of skin cancer increases your risk of developing SCC again.

5. Conditions that lower the immune system, such as HIV/AIDS or organ transplantation, or drugs that suppress the immune system, can raise the risk of developing SCC.

6. Extreme photosensitivity and an elevated risk of skin cancer are hallmarks of Xeroderma Pigmentosum, a rare genetic condition.

7. Drinking water contaminated with arsenic or occupational exposure to high amounts of arsenic both enhance the risk of skin cancer in smokers.

8. Exposure to specific chemicals and compounds, such as tar and some industrial chemicals, has been linked to an increased risk of squamous cell carcinoma.

9. The Human Papillomavirus (HPV) has been linked to an increased risk of SCC, particularly in the vaginal and anal regions, among those who have been exposed to certain strains of the virus.

10. Precancerous skin lesions, such as actinic keratosis, might increase the risk of SCC because they produce chronic inflammation of the skin.

11. Ionizing radiation exposure, such as that received during medical radiation therapy, has been linked to an increased risk of skin cancer.

12. Family History: While genetic factors may play a role, a family history of skin cancer, in general, can raise your risk.

It is crucial to recognize the potential dangers and take preventative measures. Sun safety measures include avoiding prolonged exposure to the sun, finding shade, and using sun protection products like sunscreen and protective clothes and helmets. Regular self-examinations of your skin and routine check-ups with a healthcare provider can aid with early detection and treatment if SCC does occur.

Symptoms and Indicators

Although squamous cell carcinoma (SCC) most commonly affects the skin, it can also develop in other organs where squamous cells are normally prevalent. Depending on where the tumor is located, there may be a wide range of symptoms.

Skin cancer:

• Red, scaly spots that crust over or bleed may be the first sign of SCC.

• The condition might worsen to the point where open sores or ulcers emerge and either don't heal or heal very slowly.

- Nodules or lumps that are elevated and very firm may be the first sign of SCC. These may be rough in texture and have a wart-like appearance.

- Some lesions caused by SCCs are tender or painful to the touch.

- An easily detectable indication of SCC is bleeding or crusting at the site of the lesion.

- Squamous cell carcinoma (SCC) can form inside of preexisting moles or other skin lesions, resulting in visible alterations such as enlargement, discoloration, or a change in the lesion's texture or color.

Cancer of the mouth (oral):

• Chronic Sore or Ulcer: A chronic sore or ulcer in the mouth that doesn't heal.

• Appearance of white or red spots on the tongue, lips, or inside of the mouth.

• As the tumor expands, it may restrict jaw and tongue movement, making it difficult to swallow or talk.

Cervical cancer:

• Sores or ulcers in the genital area are a common symptom of genital SCC.

• Some people may feel a burning or itchy sensation in the vaginal area.

Squamous cell carcinoma of the esophagus

• Dysphagia (difficulty swallowing) is a common symptom of esophageal SCC and can affect both solid and liquid food intake.

- Experiencing pain or discomfort in the chest is a common sensation, especially after swallowing.

- Weight loss that occurs for no apparent reason is a typical sign.

- Regurgitation: Regurgitation of food or blood may occur in more advanced situations.

It's crucial to emphasize that not all skin or oral lesions are malignant, and many skin conditions might resemble SCC. However, it's best to visit a doctor if you experience any changes to your skin's appearance or any sores that don't heal within a few weeks. In order to properly manage SCC and improve results, early identification and treatment are essential. The best course of action can be determined after a comprehensive examination, sometimes followed by a biopsy ordered by the doctor.

CHAPTER TWO
Diagnose and Classify

The prognosis and therapy of squamous cell carcinoma (SCC) depend heavily on its accurate diagnosis and staging. These steps aid in determining the tumor's extent, as well as whether or not it has spread to lymph nodes or other organs. An summary of SCC diagnosis and staging is as follows:

Diagnosis:

• First, a dermatologist or other medical professional will do a clinical evaluation. They'll take a close look at the area of skin, mucous membranes, or internal organ that has raised suspicion.

• A biopsy is usually done to confirm the diagnosis. A tissue sample from the area of concern is taken during a biopsy for further testing. Depending on the size and location of the lesion, a shave biopsy, punch biopsy, or excisional biopsy may be performed.

• Histopathological analysis involves a pathologist looking for squamous cell carcinoma cells in the biopsy sample. This analysis can also be used to determine the grade (the degree of abnormality) of the cancer cells and whether or not they have spread to deeper layers of tissue.

Tumor, lymph node, and metastasis (TNM) staging is a commonly used approach for assessing the cancer's progression and severity. Roman numerals (I, II, III, or IV) designate the stage, which may have subdivisions (e.g., stage IIa, IIb). The best course of treatment can be decided upon after the results of the staging process have been analyzed.

This is how the TNM classification for SCC works in brief:

• Primary tumor (T) size and distribution is described. There may be no primary tumor present (T stage 0) or a big tumor with widespread invasion (T stage 4).

• Whether or not the malignancy has progressed to the lymph nodes is represented by the letter N. The cancer has not migrated to any regional lymph nodes (N0) and may have spread to N3 (many or far-flung lymph nodes) in the third N stage.

• If the cancer has spread to other organs or tissues, this is indicated by the letter "M," for metastasis. Both no distant metastasis, or M0, and distant metastasis, or M1, are considered to be M stages.

Additional criteria, such as tumor grade, cancer cell characteristics, and primary tumor site, may be involved in the complicated process of SCC staging. Overall stage is calculated by adding up T, N, M, and other parameters and is used to direct treatment.

It is important to work closely with your healthcare team to understand your specific situation and the proper treatment options, as the specific staging method and terminology may vary slightly based on the site of the SCC (e.g., skin, mouth, esophagus). Depending on the extent and location of the disease, SCC can be treated with a variety of approaches, including surgery, radiation treatment, chemotherapy, immunotherapy, and targeted therapy.

Choices in Medical Care

Squamous cell carcinoma (SCC) treatment options might change based on a number of circumstances, including the cancer's stage, the tumor's location, and the patient's general condition. The following methods, or a combination of them, may be used in treatment:

1. Surgery:

• When superficial cell carcinoma (SCC) is confined to a small region of skin or mucous membrane, excision (surgical removal of the tumor and some healthy tissue around it) may be an option.

• In cases of high risk or recurrent SCC, a specialist surgical approach known as Mohs surgery may be recommended. In order to remove all cancer cells while keeping as much healthy tissue as possible, tiny layers of tissue are taken and examined under a microscope.

2. Atomic Radiation Therapy:

• Tumors are targeted with high-powered X-rays in a process called external beam radiation therapy. When surgical removal of a tumor would be too risky or impossible, this method is often utilized.

• **Brachytherapy:** In this form of radiation therapy, radioactive sources are inserted into or around the tumor.

3. Creams and ointments containing chemotherapeutic medicines or immune response modifiers may be recommended for minor, superficial skin SCCs.

4. Cryotherapy: freezing and destroying tiny SCC lesions, including actinic keratoses, with liquid nitrogen.

5. Electrodesiccation and Curettage (EDC): This treatment includes scraping away the tumor and then using an electric needle to eliminate any leftover cancer cells. It is typically reserved for tiny, non-threatening SCCs.

6. In photodynamic therapy (PDT), a photosensitizing chemical is first applied to the skin, and then the area is exposed to light. Using this method, cancer cells can be eliminated with minimal collateral injury to healthy tissue.

7. Systemic chemotherapy, which includes oral and injectable medicines, may be used to treat patients with advanced or metastatic SCC.

8. Some patients with advanced SCC may benefit from immunotherapy using immune checkpoint inhibitors or other medications that stimulate the immune system to attack cancer cells.

9. Targeted Therapy: In some situations of advanced SCC, targeted therapy medications may be utilized to selectively target the genetic mutations or abnormalities present in the cancer cells.

10. After SCC excision, reconstructive surgery may be required to restore form and function if a significant quantity of healthy tissue had to be removed.

Treatment options are determined on the type and stage of cancer present, as well as the patient's general health. Furthermore, the location of the SCC (e.g., skin, oral cavity, esophagus, genital area) may influence the course of treatment. A healthcare team, which may consist of dermatologists, surgeons, oncologists, and radiation therapists, should be consulted in order to establish the best course of treatment for each particular patient. The greatest possible outcomes for SCC are typically achieved through early detection and treatment.

CHAPTER THREE
Prediction and Treatment

The stage of the cancer, its location, the patient's overall health, and the treatment technique all play a role in the management and prognosis of squamous cell carcinoma (SCC). An outline of the treatment for SCC and its expected outcome follows.

Management:

• Squamous cell carcinoma (SCC) treatment may include one or more of the following procedures: surgery, radiation therapy, chemotherapy, immunotherapy, targeted therapy, or other specialist procedures. Treatment options are determined by the cancer's stage, its location, and the patient's preferences and health status.

• After a patient's treatment is complete, they will often have follow-up meetings with their healthcare team to check on their progress and look for any new SCCs. Follow-up care may include a skin inspection and other diagnostic procedures.

• Preventing further skin damage and lowering the risk of new SCCs is the primary goal of sun protection measures, such as sunscreen, protective clothing, sunglasses, and seeking shade, for people with a history of SCC or those at high risk.

• Patients who smoke or drink heavily are sometimes advised to make changes to their lifestyle, such as quitting smoking or cutting back on alcohol consumption, in order to lower their risk of SCC returning.

• A balanced diet and regular physical activity are important components of a healthy lifestyle that can promote general well-being and may lower the chance of cancer recurrence.

Prognosis:

The outlook for SCC varies greatly from case to case.

• The prognosis for SCC improves with earlier diagnosis and treatment. Most skin cancers have a good prognosis if they are found only on the skin's surface or in the mucous membranes. However, the prognosis is not as bright for SCCs that have penetrated deeper tissues or spread to lymph nodes or other organs.

• Prognosis is also affected by where the SCC is located. When compared to SCCs of the mouth, esophagus, or other internal organs, the prognosis for cutaneous SCCs is often better, especially if they are caught early.

• Considerable consideration must be given to the tumor's size and depth. Tumors that are smaller and less deeply rooted tend to have a better prognosis.

• The prognosis of cancer patients might be affected by the histological grade of their cancer cells. Well-differentiated SCCs (cells that closely resemble normal cells) may have a better prognosis than poorly differentiated ones.

- **Patient Health:** The patient's general health and response to treatment can have an effect on prognosis. Patients who already suffer from additional health issues may have a more difficult prognosis.

- In some cases, the prognosis may be negatively impacted by a recurrence of SCC (i.e., the disease returning after first treatment).

It's crucial to emphasize that SCC is generally curable when diagnosed and treated early, and many persons with SCC have a great prognosis. But results are not always predictable, and certain circumstances can be more difficult to handle than others. Your healthcare team is in the best position to advise you on your prognosis and treatment options given the unique circumstances of your case.

Safety and Security Measures

Squamous cell carcinoma (SCC) can be prevented and its effects lessened via careful attention to both. Some measures and habits can be taken to lessen the likelihood of developing SCC:

1. UV Blocking:

• Even on cloudy days, it's important to use a broad-spectrum sunscreen with at least an SPF of 30 on any exposed skin. Apply again every two hours, or more often if you swim or perspire heavily.

• Wearing protective clothing, such as a broad-brimmed hat, long-sleeved shirt, long pants, and sunglasses, can help prevent sun damage to your skin and eyes.

Keep out of the direct sunlight as much as possible, especially between the hours of 10 a.m. and 4 p.m.

Artificial tanning beds are dangerous because of the ultraviolet (UV) radiation they release.

2. Routine Skin Checks:

• Keep an eye out for moles, growths, and other skin anomalies by performing regular self-exams. If you detect anything unusual, consult a dermatologist for a professional review.

3. Keep Lips Safe:

• If you spend a lot of time outside, it's important to use a lip balm with SPF to prevent UV damage.

4. Stay away from Dangerous Things:

• Avoid becoming sunburned or sunbathing in the sun, both of which might increase your risk of skin cancer.

5. Avoid dehydration:

• In order to aid your skin in healing from sun exposure, it is important to stay hydrated, especially when the temperature outside is high.

6. Precautions to Take Before Working Outside:

• Those working outside should take particular care to protect themselves from the elements by using protective gear, applying sunscreen, and drinking enough of water.

7. Quitting Smoking:

• If you smoke, you can lower your chance of SCC and other health problems by giving up the habit.

8. Moderation in Alcohol Use:

• Keep your alcohol intake in check, as doing so, especially when combined with other risk factors, can raise your risk of SCC.

9. Preventative Health Care:

• If you are at risk for skin cancer or have a family history of the disease, see your doctor often for examinations.

10. Seek immediate medical assistance for any skin changes you find worrisome, such as new or changing moles or sores that won't heal. Early identification and treatment can improve the prognosis.

11. Vaccination Against Human Papillomavirus:

• Human papillomavirus (HPV) vaccine may be recommended to lower the risk of developing genital and oral SCC.

12. Visits to the Dentist Twice a Year

• If you want to avoid developing oral SCC, it's important to practice good oral hygiene and get frequent dental checkups. This can aid in the early detection and resolution of problems.

13. A Healthy Esophagus

• To reduce your risk of developing esophageal SCC, you should limit your intake of alcoholic beverages and tobacco products, eat a healthy, balanced diet, and contact a doctor if you have chronic problems swallowing.

You can lessen your chances of developing squamous cell carcinoma by adopting these preventative practices and adjusting your lifestyle accordingly. You can reduce your chance of SCC and other skin cancers by taking preventative measures including wearing sunscreen, going in for frequent checkups, and adopting a healthy lifestyle.

CHAPTER FOUR
Adjusting to a New Health Status

It can be difficult and upsetting to learn that you have squamous cell carcinoma (SCC) or any other type of cancer. The emotional and practical components of dealing with a cancer diagnosis are equally important. If you or a loved one has been diagnosed with SCC, here are some ways to deal with the news.

1. Ask for Help:

• If you need someone to talk to, call, or text a loved one. Don't hesitate to communicate your sentiments and concerns with loved ones.

Join a cancer support group or look for individuals who have been through what you're going through. These gatherings facilitate the sharing of personal stories and the provision of emotional solace.

2. Learn Something:

• You should study up on SCC to familiarize yourself with the disease and its possible outcomes. Fear and worry might be lessened by learning as much as you can about your situation.

3. Get in Touch with Your Doctor:

• Communicate effectively and openly with your medical staff. Ask questions, seek clarification, and share your concerns and wishes.

4. Grasp the Facts and Move Forward

• Work together with your healthcare team to discuss your treatment options in detail. If you're still not sure, you might want to get a second opinion.

5. Wellness in Mind and Heart

• Think about seeing a therapist or counselor to help you cope with the diagnosis's emotional toll.

Stress and anxiety may be alleviated by practices like yoga, meditation, and mindfulness training.

6. Observe a Healthy Way of Life:

• Maintain a healthy lifestyle by sticking to a balanced diet, working out regularly as directed by your healthcare providers, and getting plenty of rest.

7. If you want to get better, you need to do what the doctor says.

Take responsibility for your own health and well-being by attending to things like managing treatment-related side effects, taking prescribed medications, and practicing excellent hygiene.

8. Share Your Feelings:

• Maintain a notebook in which you can write down your feelings and thoughts. Journaling is a healthy approach to record your thoughts and feelings as well as keep track of your progress.

9. Rely on Your Friends and Family:

Having friends and family help out with mundane tasks like errand running and meal preparation may be a huge stress reliever.

10. Attempt to Achieve Only Reasonable Objectives

• Make plans for your future that you can actually achieve, and reward yourself when you do.

11. Think about having a conversation with your healthcare team and loved ones about your long-term goals, including your wishes regarding end-of-life care.

12. Check Out Alternative Treatments:

• Some persons find complementary therapies, such as acupuncture, massage, or art therapy, effective for managing symptoms and enhancing well-being.

13. Educate yourself:

• Keep up with the latest findings and therapies for SCC. You can gain strength and confidence through education.

14. Try to Keep a Good Mood:

• Keep a good disposition and worry about things you can change. Put oneself in an optimistic environment.

Remember that coping with a cancer diagnosis is a personal journey, and everyone's experience is different. It's crucial to look for the help and materials that are a good fit for you. Throughout your experience with SCC, don't be afraid to ask for help from your healthcare team. They can help you deal with your diagnosis and treatment by giving you information, resources, and referrals.

Conclusion

Squamous cell carcinoma (SCC) is a frequent kind of cancer that can manifest anywhere, including the skin, mucous membranes, and internal organs. Factors like sun exposure, pale skin, and certain lifestyle choices have been linked to an increased chance of developing this condition. The key to successful early discovery and management of SCC is knowledge of its symptoms, diagnosis, and available treatments.

• The risk of SCC can be reduced with sun protection, self-examinations, and maintaining a healthy lifestyle. If diagnosed with

SCC, obtaining medical attention and implementing a treatment plan specific to the particular case are crucial steps in improving the prognosis.

- There are both mental and physical steps to take after learning of a cancer diagnosis like SCC. These include reaching out to others, learning as much as possible, and keeping an optimistic attitude. Diagnosis and treatment can be a long and winding road, but with the correct help, knowledge, and forethought, anyone can travel it.

The good news is that with early detection and continued research and improvement in the field of cancer treatment, SCC is often efficiently controlled. One of the most important aspects of dealing with SCC and other health difficulties is getting the advice and support of medical professionals and loved ones.

THE END